Keto Diet Cookbook For Beginners

Delicious, fast and healthy recipes

Sommario

INTRODUCTION

Hi everyone, I'm glad and proud that you're here to improve your nutritional style, that's why I created this awesome cookbook with the best recipes for the first half of the day! Breakfast and lunch are the most important meals of the day, the meals where the energy intake must be the highest. Here you will find quick and easy recipes full of protein, taste and vitamins.

But let's not get lost in too many words, and start cooking together....

DINNER

CHEESY SALMON & ASPARAGUS

Ingredients:

- 4 Salmon Fillets, 6 Ounces Each & Skin On

- 2 lbs. Asparagus, Trimmed

- 6 Tablespoons Butter

- 4 Cloves Garlic, Minced

- ½ Cup Parmesan Cheese, Grated

- Sea Salt & Black Pepper to Taste

Instructions

1. Start by heating your oven to 400, lining a baking sheet with foil.

2. Pat your salmon dry, seasoning with salt and pepper.

3. Put your salmon in a pan, arranging your asparagus around it.

4. Put a saucepan over medium heat and melt your butter. Add in your garlic, stirring until it browns which takes about three minutes. Drizzle this butter over your salmon and asparagus.

5. Top with parmesan cheese and then cook for twelve minutes. Broil for another three before serving warm.

Preparation Time: 15 minutes **Servings:** 4

Cooking Time: 15 Minutes

Nutrition: Calories: 434 Protein: 42g Fat: 26g Net Carbs: 6g

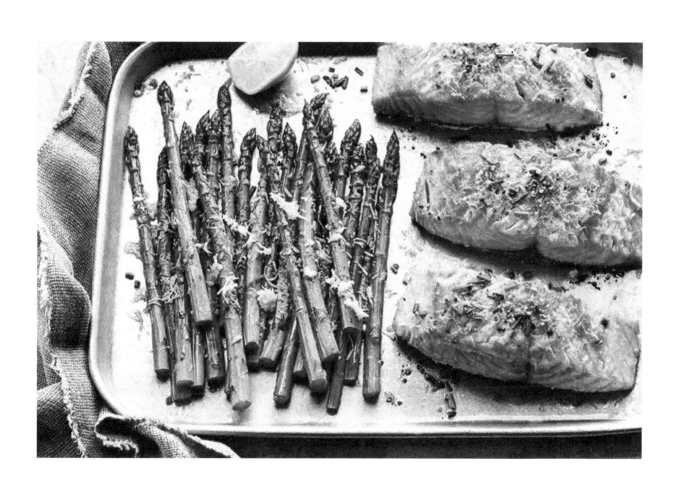

HERB PORK CHOPS

Ingredients:

- 2 Tablespoons Butter + More for Coating

- 4 Pork Chops, Boneless

- 2 Tablespoons Italian Seasoning

- 2 Tablespoons Italian Leaf Parsley Chopped

- 2 Tablespoons Olive Oil

- Sea Salt & Black Pepper to Taste

Instructions

1. Start by heating your oven to 350 and coat a baking dish with butter.

2. Season your pork chops, and then top with fresh parsley, drizzling with olive oil and a half a tablespoon of butter each to bake.

3. Bake for twenty to twenty-five minutes.

Preparation Time: minutes **Servings:** 4

Cooking Time: 30 Minutes

Nutrition: Calories: 333 Protein: 31g Fat: 23g Net Carbs: 0g

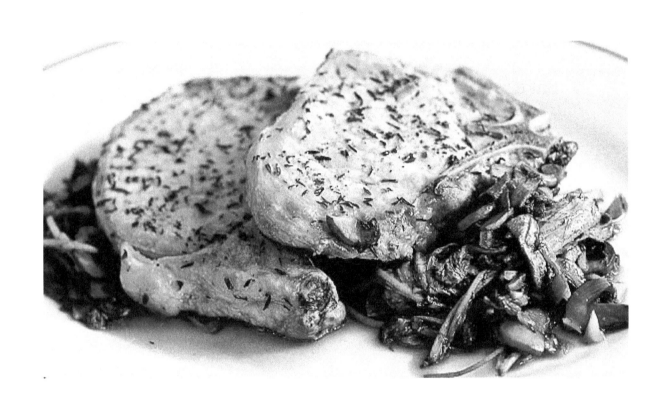

PAPRIKA CHICKEN

Ingredients:

- 2 Teaspoons Smoked Paprika

- ½ Cup Heavy Whipping Cream

- ½ Cup Sweet Onion, Chopped

- 1 Tablespoon Olive Oil

- 4 Chicken Breasts, Skin On & 4 Ounces Each

- ½ Cup Sour Cream

- 2 Tablespoons Parsley, Chopped

Instructions

1. Season your chicken with salt and pepper, putting a skillet over medium-high heat. Add your oil, and once it simmers, sear your chicken on both sides. It should take about fifteen minutes to cook your chicken all the way through. Put your chicken to the side.

2. Add in your onion, sautéing for four minutes or until tender.

3. Stir in your paprika and cream, bringing it to a simmer.

4. Return your chicken to the skillet, simmering for five more minutes.

5. Stir in sour cream and serve topped with parsley.

Preparation Time: 15 minutes **Servings:** 4

Cooking Time: 20 Minutes

Nutrition: Calories: 389 Protein: 25gFat: 30g Net Carbs: 4g

COCONUT CHICKEN

Ingredients:

- 1 Teaspoon Ground Cumin

- 1 Teaspoon Ground Coriander

- ¼ Cup Cilantro, Fresh & Chopped

- 1 Cup Coconut Milk

- 1 Tablespoon Curry Powder

- ½ Cup Sweet Onion, Chopped

- 2 Tablespoons Olive Oil

- 4 Chicken Breasts, 4 Ounces Each & Cut into 2 Inch Chunks

Instructions

1. Get out a saucepan, adding in your oil and heating it over medium-high heat.

2. Sauté your chicken until it's almost completely cooked, which will take roughly ten minutes.

3. Add in your onion, cooking for another three minutes.

4. Whisk your curry powder, coconut milk, coriander and cumin together.

5. Pour the sauce into your pan, bringing it to a boil with your chicken.

6. Reduce the heat, and let it simmer for ten minutes.

7. Serve topped with cilantro.

Preparation Time: 10 minutes **Servings:** 4

Cooking Time: 30 Minutes

Nutrition: Calories: 382 Protein: 23g Fat: 31g Net Carbs: 4g

CABBAGE & CHICKEN PLATES

Ingredients:

- 1 Cup Bean Sprouts, Fresh

- 2 Tablespoons Sesame & Garlic Flavored Oil

- ½ Cup Onion, Sliced

- 4 Cups Bok Choy, Shredded

- 3 Stalks Celery, Chopped

- 1 Tablespoon Ginger, Minced

- 2 Tablespoon Coconut Aminos

- 1 Teaspoon Stevia

- 1 Cup Chicken Broth

- 1 ½ Teaspoons Minced Garlic

- 1 Teaspoon Arrowroot

- 4 Chicken Breasts, Boneless, Cooked & Sliced Thin

Instructions

1. Shred your cabbage, and then add your chicken and onion together.

2. Add in a dollop of mayonnaise if desired, drizzling with oil

3. Season as desired and serve.

Preparation Time: 25 minutes **Servings:** 4

Cooking Time: 0 Minutes

Nutrition: Calories: 368 Protein: 42g Fat: 18g Net Carbs: 8g

GRILLED CHICKEN & CHEESY SPINACH

Ingredients:

- 3 Ounces Mozzarella Cheese, Part Skim

- 3 Chicken Breasts, Large & Sliced in Half

- 10 Ounces Spinach, Frozen, Thawed & Drained

- ½ Cup Roasted Red Peppers, Sliced into Strips

- 2 Cloves Garlic Minced

- 1 Teaspoon Olive Oil

- Sea Salt & Black Pepper to Taste

Instructions

1. Start by heating your oven to 400, and then grease a pan.

2. Bake your chicken breasts for two to three minutes per side.

3. In another skillet, cook your garlic and spinach in oil for three minutes.

4. Put your chicken on a pan, topping it with spinach, roasted peppers and mozzarella.

5. Bake until your cheese melts and serve warm.

Preparation Time: 7minutes **Servings:** 6

Cooking Time: 6 Minutes

Nutrition: Calories: 195 Protein: 30g Fat: 7g Net Carbs: 3g

BALSAMIC CHICKEN WITH VEGETABLES

Ingredients:

- 8 chicken Cutlets, Skinless & Boneless

- ½ Cup Buttermilk, Low Fat

- 4 Tablespoons Dijon Mustard

- 2/3 Cup Almond Meal

- 2/3 Cup Cashews Chopped

- 4 Teaspoons Stevia

- ¾ Teaspoon Rosemary

- Sea Salt & Black Pepper to Taste

Instructions

1. Start by heating your oven to 425.

2. Mix your buttermilk and mustard together in a bowl

3. Add your chicken, coating it.

4. Put a skillet over medium heat, and then add in your almond meal. Bake until its golden, putting it in a bowl.

5. Add your sea salt, pepper, rosemary and cashews, mixing well. Coat your chicken with the almond meal mix, and then put it in a baking pan.

6. Bake for twenty-five minutes.

Preparation Time: 15 minutes **Servings:** 4

Cooking Time: 25 Minutes

Nutrition: Calories: 248 Protein: 27g Fat: 8g Net Carbs: 14g

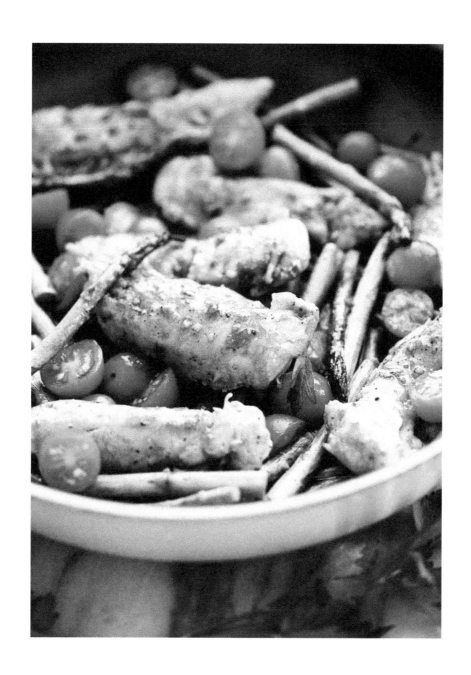

STEAK & BROCCOLI MEDLEY

Ingredients:

- 4 Ounces Butter

- ¾ lb. Ribeye Steak

- 9 Ounces Broccoli

- 1 Yellow Onion

- 1 Tablespoon Coconut Aminos

- 1 Tablespoon Pumpkin Seeds

- Sea Salt & Black Pepper as Needed

Instructions

1. Slice your onion and steak before chopping your broccoli.

2. Put a frying pan over medium heat, adding in butter. Let it melt, and then add meat. Season with salt and pepper, placing your meat to the side.

3. Brown your onion and broccoli, adding more butter as necessary.

4. Add in your coconut aminos before adding your meat back.

5. Serve topped with pumpkin seeds and butter.

Preparation Time: 10 minutes **Servings:** 4

Cooking Time: 10 Minutes

Nutrition: Calories: 875 Protein: 40g Fat: 75g Net Carbs: 10g

STUFFED MEAT LOAF

Ingredients:

- 17 Ounces Ground Beef

- ¼ Cup Onions, Diced

- 6 Slices Cheddar Cheese

- ¼ Cup Green Onions, Diced

- ½ Cup Spinach

- ¼ Cup Mushrooms

Instructions

- Mix your salt, pepper, meat, cumin and garlic together before greasing a pan.

- Put your cheese on the bottom of your meatloaf, adding in the spinach, mushrooms and onions, and then use leftover meat to cover the top.

- Bake at 350 for an hour before serving.

Preparation Time: 20 minutes **Servings:** 8

Cooking Time: 1 Hour

Nutrition: Calories: 248 Protein: 15g Fat: 20g Net Carbs: 1g

BEEF CABBAGE ROLLS

Ingredients:

- 3 ½ lb. Corned Beef

- 15 Cabbage Leaves, Large

- 1 Onion

- 1 Lemon

- ¼ Cup Coffee

- ¼ Cup White Wine

- 1 Tablespoon Bacon Fat, Rendered

- 1 Tablespoon Brown Mustard

- 2 Tablespoons Himalayan Pink Sea Salt

- 2 Tablespoons Worcestershire Sauce

- 1 Teaspoon Whole Peppercorns

- 1 Teaspoon Mustard Seeds

- ½ Teaspoon Red Pepper Flakes

- ¼ Teaspoons Cloves

- ¼ Teaspoon Allspice

- 1 Bay Leaf, Large

Instructions

1. Add your liquids, corned beef and spices into a slow cooker, cooking on low for six hours.

2. Bring a pot of water to a boil, adding your cabbage leaves and one sliced onion, bringing it to a boil for three minutes.

3. Remove your cabbage, putting it in ice water for three to four minutes, continuing to boil your onion.

4. Dry the leaves off, slicing your meat, and adding in your cooked onion and meat into your leaves.

Preparation Time: 20 minutes **Servings:** 5

Cooking Time: 6 Hours 10 Minutes

Nutrition: Calories: 481 Protein: 35g Fat: 25g Net Carbs: 4g

ZUCCHINI FETTUCCINE WITH BEEF

Ingredients:

- 15 oz. ground beef

- 3 tbsp. butter

- 1 yellow onion

- 8 oz. mushrooms

- 1 tbsp. dried thyme

- ½ tsp salt

- 1 pinch ground black pepper

- 8 oz. blue cheese

- 1½ cups sour cream

Zucchini fettuccine:

- 2 zucchinis

- 1 oz. olive oil or butter

- Salt and pepper

Instructions

1. Peel the onion and chop it finely.

2. Melt the butter and sauté the onion until the onions are softened and transparent.

3. Add the ground beef and fry this for a few more minutes with the onion until it is browned and cooked through.

4. Slice or dice the mushrooms, and add it to the ground beef. Sauté the mushrooms with the beef mixture for a few minutes more, or until lightly brown.

5. Season it with thyme, salt, and pepper. Crumble the cheese over the hot mixture. Stir it well.

6. Add the sour cream and bring the mixture to a light boil. Lower the heat to a medium-low setting and let it simmer for about 10 minutes.

Zucchini fettuccine:

- Calculate about one medium-sized zucchini per person.

- Slice the zucchini lengthwise in half.

- Scoop out the seeds with a spoon and slice the halves super thinly, lengthwise (julienne) with a potato peeler, or you can use a spiralizer to make zoodles (zucchini noodles.)

- Toss the zucchini in some hot sauce of your choice and serve it immediately.

- If you are not going to be serving your zucchini with a hot sauce, then boil half a gallon of salted water in a large pot and parboil the zucchini slices for a minute. This makes them easier to eat

- Drain the water from the pot and add some olive oil or a knob of butter. Salt and pepper to taste.

Preparation Time: 15 minutes **Servings:** 4

Cooking Time: 30 minutes

Nutrition: Calories: 456 Protein: 32g Fat: 15g Net Carbs: 13g

OVEN-BAKED CHICKEN IN GARLIC BUTTER

Ingredients:

- 3 lbs. chickens, a whole bird

- 2 tsp sea salt

- ½ tsp ground black pepper

- 51/3 oz. butter

- 2 garlic cloves, minced

Instructions

1. Preheat the oven to 400°F.

2. Season the chicken with salt and pepper, both inside and out.

3. The chicken must go breast side up in the baking dish.

4. Combine the garlic and butter in a saucepan over a medium heat. The butter should not turn brown or burn, just melt it gently.

5. Let the butter cool down once it is melted.

6. Pour the garlic butter mixture all over and inside the chicken. Bake the chicken on the lower oven rack for 1 to1 ½ hours, or until internal temperature reaches 180°F. Baste it with the juices from the bottom of the pan every 20 minutes.

7. Serve with the juices.

Preparation Time: 25 minutes **Servings:** 3

Cooking Time: 1 hour 30 minutes

Nutrition: Calories: 148 Protein: 39g Fat: 24g Net Carbs: 16g

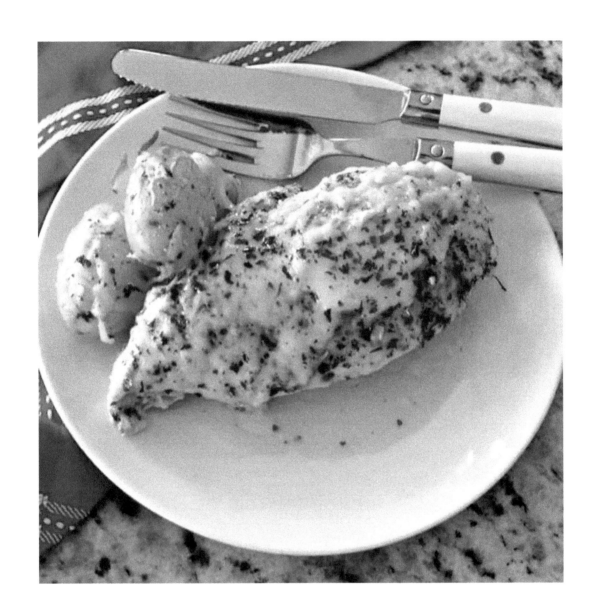

KETO CHICKEN GARAM MASALA

Ingredients:

- 25 oz. chicken breasts

- 3 tbsp. butter or ghee

- Salt

- 1 red bell pepper, finely diced

- 1¼ cups coconut cream or heavy whipping cream

- 1 tbsp. fresh parsley, finely chopped

- Garam masala:

- 1 tsp ground cumin

- 1 - 2 tsp coriander seed, ground

- 1 tsp ground cardamom (green)

- 1 tsp turmeric, ground

- 1 tsp ground ginger

- 1 tsp paprika powder

- 1 tsp chili powder

- 1 pinch ground nutmeg

Instructions

1. Preheat the oven to 400°F.

2. Mix the spices together for the Garam masala.

3. Cut the chicken breasts lengthwise. Place a large skillet over medium-high heat and fry the chicken in the butter until it is golden-brown.

4. Add half of the garam masala spice mix to the pan and stir it thoroughly.

5. Season with some salt, and place the chicken and all of the juices, into a baking dish.

6. Finely chop the bell pepper and add it to a bowl along with the coconut cream and the remaining half of the garam masala spice mix.

7. Pour over the chicken. Bake for 20 minutes.

8. Garnish with parsley and serve.

Preparation Time: 10 minutes **Servings:** 4

Cooking Time: 20 minutes

Nutrition: Calories: 312 Protein: 21g Fat: 14g Net Carbs: 2g

KETO LASAGNA

Ingredients:

- 2 tbsp. olive oil

- 1 yellow onion

- 1 garlic clove

- 20 oz. ground beef

- 3 tbsp. tomato paste

- ½ tbsp. dried basil

- 1 tsp salt

- ¼ tsp ground black pepper

- ½ cup water

- Keto pasta

- 8 eggs

- 10 oz. cream cheese

- 1 tsp salt

- 5 tbsp. ground psyllium husk powder

Cheese topping:

- 2 cups crème fraiche or sour cream

- 5 oz. shredded cheese

- 2 oz. grated parmesan cheese

- ½ tsp salt

- ¼ tsp ground black pepper

- ½ cup fresh parsley, finely chopped

Instructions

1. Start with the ground beef mixture.

2. Peel and finely chop the onion and the garlic. Fry them in olive oil until they are soft. Add the ground beef to the onion and garlic and cook until it is golden. Add the tomato paste and remaining spices.

3. Stir the mixture thoroughly and add some water. Bring it to a boil, turn the heat down, and let it simmer for at least 15 minutes, or until the majority of the water has evaporated. The lasagna sheets used don't soak up as much liquid as regular ones, so the mixture should be quite dry.

4. While that is happening, make the lasagna sheets according to the instructions that follow below.

5. Preheat the oven to 400°F. Mix the shredded cheese with sour cream and the Parmesan cheese. Reserve one or two tablespoons of the cheese aside for the topping. Add salt and pepper for taste and stir in the parsley.

6. Place the lasagna sheets and pasta sauce in layers in a greased baking dish.

7. Spread the crème fraiche mixture and the reserved Parmesan cheese on top.

8. Bake the lasagna in the oven for around 30 minutes or until the lasagna has a nicely browned surface. Serve with a green salad and a light dressing.

Lasagna sheets:

1. Preheat the oven to 300°F.

2. Add the eggs, cream cheese, and the salt to a mixing bowl and blend into a smooth batter. Continue to whisk this while adding in the ground psyllium husk powder, just a little bit at a time. Let it sit for a few minutes.

3. Using a spatula spread the batter onto a baking sheet that is lined with parchment paper. Place more parchment paper on top and flatten it with a rolling pin until the mixture is at least 13" x 18". You can also divide it into two separate batches and use a different baking sheet for even thinner pasta.

4. Let the pieces of parchment paper stay in place. Bake the pasta for about 10 to12 minutes. Let it cool and remove the paper. Slice into sheets.

Preparation Time: 25 minutes **Servings:** 4

Cooking Time: 1 hour minutes

Nutrition: Calories: 128 Protein: 25g Fat: 15g Net Carbs: 4g

KETO BUFFALO DRUMSTICKS AND CHILI AIOLI

Ingredients:

- 2 lbs. chicken drumsticks or chicken wings

- 2 tbsp. olive oil or coconut oil

- 2 tbsp. white wine vinegar

- 1 tbsp. tomato paste

- 1 tsp salt

- 1 tsp paprika powder

- 1 tablespoon Tabasco

- Butter or olive oil, for greasing the baking dish

Chili aioli:

- 2/3 cup mayonnaise

- 1 tablespoon smoked paprika powder or smoked chili powder

- 1 garlic clove, minced

Instructions

1. Preheat the oven to 450° (220°C).

2. Put the drumsticks in a plastic bag.

3. Mix the ingredients for the marinade and pour into the plastic bag. Shake the bag and let marinate for 10 minutes.

4. Coat a baking dish with oil. Place the drumsticks in the baking bowl and let bake for 30–40 minutes or until they are done and have turned a beautiful color.

5. Mix together mayonnaise, garlic, and chili.

Preparation Time: 12 minutes **Servings:** 6

Cooking Time: 40 minutes

Nutrition: Calories: 409 Protein: 22g Fat: 10g Net Carbs: 6g

KETO FISH CASSEROLE

Ingredients:

- 2 tbsp. olive oil

- 15 oz. broccoli

- 6 scallions

- 2 tbsp. small capers

- 1/6 oz. butter, for greasing the casserole dish

- 25 oz. white fish, in serving-sized pieces

- 1¼ cups heavy whipping cream

- 1 tbsp. Dijon mustard

- 1 tsp salt

- ¼ tsp ground black pepper

- 1 tbsp. dried parsley

- 3 oz. butter

Instructions

1. Preheat the oven to 400°F.

2. Divide the broccoli into smaller floret heads and include the stems. Peel it with a sharp knife or a potato peeler if the stem is rough or leafy.

3. Fry the broccoli florets in oil on a medium-high heat for about 5 minutes, until they are golden and soft. Season with salt and pepper to taste.

4. Add finely chopped scallions and the capers. Fry this for another 1 to 2 minutes and place the vegetables in a baking dish that has been greased.

5. Place the fish tightly in amongst the vegetables.

6. Mix the parsley, whipping cream and mustard together. Pour this over the fish and vegetables. Top it with slices of butter.

7. Bake the fish until it is cooked through, and it flakes easily with a fork. Serve as is, or with a tasty green salad.

Preparation Time: 10 minutes **Servings:** 4

Cooking Time: 20 minutes

Nutrition: Calories: 314 Protein: 20g Fat: 8g Net Carbs: 5g

SLOW COOKER KETO PORK ROAST

Ingredients:

- 30 oz. pork shoulder or pork roast

- ½ tbsp. salt

- 1 bay leaf

- 5 black peppercorns

- 2½ cups water

- 2 tsp dried thyme or dried rosemary

- 2 garlic cloves

- 1½ oz. fresh ginger

- 1 tbsp. olive oil or coconut oil

- 1 tbsp. paprika powder

- ½ tsp ground black pepper

Creamy gravy:

- 1½ cups heavy whipping cream

- Juices from the roast

Instructions

1. Preheat the oven to a low heat of 200°F.

2. Season the meat with salt and place it into a deep baking dish.

3. Add water. Add a bay leaf, peppercorns, and thyme for more seasoning. Place the baking bowl in the oven for 7 to 8 hours and cover it with aluminum foil.

4. If you are using a slow cooker for this, do the same process as in step 2, only add 1 cup of water. Cook it for 8 hours on low or for 4 hours on high setting.

5. Take the meat out of the baking dish, and reserve the pan juices in a separate pan to make gravy.

6. Turn the oven up to 450°F.

7. Finely chop or press the garlic and ginger into a small bowl. Add the oil, herbs, and pepper and stir well to combine together.

8. Rub the meat with the garlic and herb mixture.

9. Return the meat back to the baking dish, and roast it for about 10 to 15 minutes or until it looks golden-brown.

10. Cut the meat into thin slices to serve it with the creamy gravy and a fibrous vegetable side dish

Gravy:

- Strain the reserved pan juices to get rid of any solid pieces from the liquid. Boil and reduce the pan juices to about half the original volume, this should be about 1 cup.

- Pour the reduction into a pot with the whipping cream. Bring this to a boil. Reduce the heat and let it simmer to your desired consistency for a creamy gravy.

Preparation Time: 35 minutes **Servings:** 4

Cooking Time: 8 hours 20 minutes

Nutrition: Calories: 432 Protein: 15g Fat: 29g Net Carbs: 13g

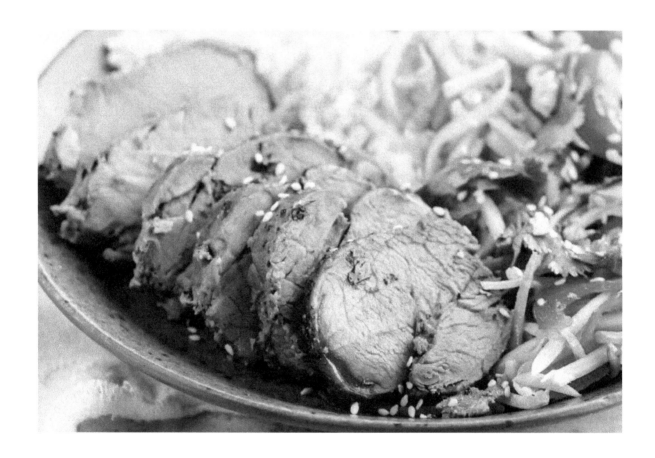

FRIED EGGS WITH KALE AND PORK

Ingredients:

- ½ lb. kale

- 3 oz. butter

- 6 oz. smoked pork belly or bacon

- ¼ cup frozen cranberries

- 1 oz. pecans or walnuts

- 4 eggs

- Salt and pepper

Instructions

1. Cut and chop the kale into large squares. You can use pre-washed baby kale as a shortcut if you want. Melt two-thirds of the butter in a frying pan, and fry the kale on high heat until it is slightly browned around its edges.

2. Remove the kale from the frying pan and put it aside. Sear the pork belly in the same frying pan until it is crispy.

3. Turn the heat down. Put the sautéed kale back into the pan and add the cranberries and nuts. Stir this mixture until it is warmed through. Put it into a bowl on the side.

4. Turn up the heat once more, and fry the eggs in the remaining amount of the butter. Add salt and pepper to taste. Serve the eggs and greens immediately.

Preparation Time: 15 minutes **Servings:** 5

Cooking Time: 20 minutes

Nutrition: Calories: 180 Protein: 23g Fat: 30g Net Carbs: 13g

CAULIFLOWER SOUP WITH PANCETTA

Ingredients:

- 4 cups chicken broth or vegetable stock

- 15 oz. cauliflower

- 7 oz. cream cheese

- 1 tbsp. Dijon mustard

- 4 oz. butter

- Salt and pepper

- 7 oz. pancetta or bacon, diced

- 1 tbsp. butter, for frying

- 1 teaspoon paprika powder or smoked chili powder

- 3 oz. pecans

Instructions

1. Trim the cauliflower and cut it into smaller floret heads. The smaller the florets are, the quicker the soup will be ready.

2. Put aside a handful of the fresh cauliflower and chop into small 1/4 inch bits.

3. Sauté the finely chopped cauliflower and pancetta in butter until it is crispy. Add some nuts and the paprika powder at the end. Set aside the mixture for serving.

4. Boil the cauliflower until they are soft. Add the cream cheese, mustard, and butter.

5. Stir the soup well, using an immersion blender, to get to the desired consistency. The creamier the soup will become the longer you blend. Salt and pepper the soup to taste.

6. Serve soup in bowls, and top it with the fried pancetta mixture.

Preparation Time: 15 minutes **Servings:** 4

Cooking Time: 35 minutes

Nutrition: Calories: 112 Protein: 10g Fat: 22g Net Carbs: 21g

BUTTER MAYONNAISE

Ingredients:

- 51/3 oz. butter

- 1 egg yolk

- 1 tbsp. Dijon mustard

- 1 tsp lemon juice

- ¼ tsp salt

- 1 pinch ground black pepper

Instructions

- Melt the butter in a small saucepan. Pour it into a small pitcher or a jug with a spout and let the butter cool.

- Mix together egg yolks and mustard in a small-sized bowl. Pour the butter in a thin stream while beating it with a hand mixer. Leave the sediment that settles at the bottom.

- Keep beating the mixture until the mayonnaise turns thick and creamy. Add some lemon juice. Season it with salt and black pepper. Serve this immediately.

Preparation Time: 20 minutes **Servings:** 4

Cooking Time: 25 minutes

Nutrition: Calories: 428 Protein: 45g Fat: 4g Net Carbs: 14g

MEATLOAF WRAPPED IN BACON

Ingredients:

- 2 tbsp. butter

- 1 yellow onion, finely chopped

- 25 oz. ground beef or ground lamb/pork

- ½ cup heavy whipping cream

- ½ cup shredded cheese

- 1 egg

- 1 tbsp. dried oregano or dried basil

- 1 tsp salt

- ½ tsp ground black pepper

- 7 oz. sliced bacon

- 1¼ cups heavy whipping cream, for the gravy

Instructions

- Preheat the oven to 400°F.

- Fry the onion until it is soft but not overly browned.

- Mix the ground meat in a bowl with all the other ingredients, minus the bacon. Mix it well, but avoid overworking it as you do not want the mixture to become dense.

- Mold the meat into a loaf shape and place it in a baking dish. Wrap the loaf completely in the bacon.

- Bake the loaf in the middle rack of the oven for about 45 minutes. If you notice that the bacon begins to overcook before the meat is done, cover it with some aluminum foil and lower the heat a bit since you do not want burnt bacon.

- Save all the juices that have accumulated in the baking dish from the meat and bacon, and use to make the gravy. Mix these juices and the cream in a smaller saucepan for the gravy.

- Bring it to a boil and lower the heat and let it simmer for 10 to 15 minutes until it has the right consistency and is not lumpy.

- Serve the meatloaf.

- Serve with freshly boiled broccoli or some cauliflower with butter, salt, and pepper.

Preparation Time: 10 minutes **Servings:** 3

Cooking Time: 15 minutes

Nutrition: Calories: 308 Protein: 21g Fat: 8g Net Carbs: 19g

KETO SALMON WITH BROCCOLI MASH

Ingredients:

Salmon burgers:

- 1½ lbs. salmon

- 1 egg

- ½ yellow onion

- 1 tsp salt

- ½ tsp pepper

- 2 oz. butter, for frying

- Green mash

- 1 lb. broccoli

- 5 oz. butter

- 2 oz. grated parmesan

- Salt and pepper

Lemon butter:

- 4 oz. butter at room temperature

- 2 tablespoons lemon juice

- Salt and pepper to taste

Instructions

1. Preheat the oven to 220° F. Cut the fish into smaller pieces and place them along with the rest of the ingredients for the burger, into a food processor.

2. Blend it for 30 to 45 seconds until you have a rough mixture. Don't mix it too thoroughly as you do not want tough burgers.

3. Shape 6 to 8 burgers and fry them for 4 to 5 minutes on each side on a medium heat in a generous amount of butter. Or even oil if you prefer. Keep them warm in the oven.

4. Trim the broccoli and cut it into smaller florets. You can use the stems as well just peel them and chop it into small pieces.

5. Bring a pot of salted water to a boil and add the broccoli to this. Cook it for a few minutes until it is soft, but not until all the texture is gone. Drain and discard the water used for boiling.

6. Use an immersion blender or even a food processor to mix the broccoli with the butter and the parmesan cheese. Season the broccoli mash to taste with salt and pepper.

7. Make the lemon butter by mixing room temperature butter with lemon juice, salt and pepper into a small bowl using electric beaters.

8. Serve the warm burgers with the side of green broccoli mash and a melting dollop of fresh lemon butter on top of the burger.

Preparation Time: 20 minutes **Servings:** 5

Cooking Time: 15 minutes

Nutrition: Calories: 156 Protein: 15g Fat: 11g Net Carbs: 5g

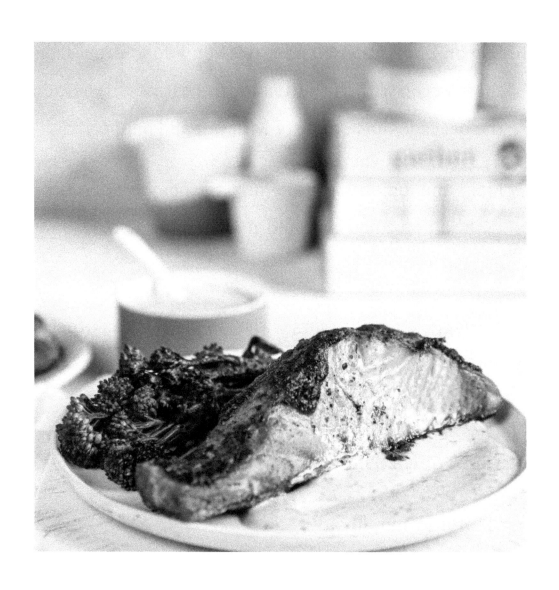

OVEN BAKED SAUSAGE AND VEGETABLES

Ingredients:

- 1 oz. butter, for greasing the baking dish

- 1 small zucchini

- 2 yellow onions

- 3 garlic cloves

- 51/3 oz. tomatoes

- 7 oz. fresh mozzarella

- Sea salt

- Black pepper

- 1 tbsp. dried basil

- Olive oil

- 1 lb. sausages in links, in links

For Servings:

- 1/2 cup mayonnaise

Instructions

1. Preheat the oven to 400°F. Grease the baking dish with butter.

2. Divide the zucchini into bite-sized pieces. Peel and cut the onion into wedges. Slice or chop the garlic.

3. Place zucchini, onions, garlic, and tomatoes in the baking dish. Dice the cheese and place among the vegetables. Season with salt, pepper and basil.

4. Sprinkle olive oil over the vegetables, and top with sausage.

5. Bake until the sausages are thoroughly cooked and the vegetables are browned.

6. Serve with a dollop of mayonnaise.

Preparation Time: 10 minutes **Servings:** 2

Cooking Time: 25 minutes

Nutrition: Calories: 176 Protein: 31g Fat: 12g Net Carbs: 10g

KETO AVOCADO QUICHE

Ingredients:

- Pie crust

- ¾ cup almond flour

- 4 tbsp. sesame seeds

- 4 tbsp. coconut flour

- 1 tbsp. ground psyllium husk powder

- 1 tsp baking powder

- 1 pinch salt

- 3 tbsp. olive oil or coconut oil

- 1 egg

- 4 tbsp. water

Filling:

- 2 avocados, ripe

- Mayonnaise

- 3 eggs

- 2tbspfinely chopped fresh cilantro

- 1 finely chopped red chili

- Onion powder

- Salt

- ½ cup cream cheese

- 1¼ cups shredded cheese

Instructions

1. Preheat the oven to 350° F. Mix all the ingredients together for the pie dough in a food processor until the dough forms into a ball, this takes a few minutes usually. Use your hands or a fork in the absence of a food processor to knead the dough together.

2. Place a piece of parchment paper to a springform pan, no larger than 12 inches around. The springform pan makes it easier to take the pie out when it is done. Grease the pan and the parchment paper.

3. Using an oiled spatula or oil coated fingers, spread the dough into the pan. Bake the crust for 10 minutes.

4. Split the avocado in half. Remove the peel and pit it, and dice the avocado.

5. Take the seeds out from the chili and chop the chili very finely. Combine the avocado and the chili in a bowl and mix them together with the other ingredients.

6. Pour the mixture into the pie crust and bake it for 35 minutes or until it is a light golden brown. Serve it with a green salad.

Preparation Time: 15 minutes **Servings:** 4

Cooking Time: 10 minutes

Nutrition: Calories: 323 Protein: 45g Fat: 18g Net Carbs: 10g

KETO BERRY MOUSSE

Ingredients:

- 2 cups heavy whipping cream

- 3 oz. fresh raspberries, strawberries or even blueberries

- 2 oz. chopped pecans

- ½ lemon the zest

- ¼ tsp vanilla extract

Instructions

1. Pour the cream into a bowl and whip it with a hand mixer until soft peaks form. You can use an old whip too, but this will take some time. Add the lemon zest and vanilla once you are almost done whipping the cream mixture.

2. Combine berries and nuts into the whipped cream and stir it thoroughly.

3. Cover the mousse with plastic wrap and let it sit in the refrigerator for 3 or more hours for a firmer mousse. If your

goal is to have a less firm consistency, you can eat the dessert right away.

Preparation Time: 10 minutes **Servings:** 4

Cooking Time: 20 minutes

Nutrition: Calories: 105 Protein: 33g Fat: 14g Net Carbs: 20g

CINNAMON CRUNCH BALLS

Ingredients:

- Unsalted butter

- Unsweetened shredded coconut

- Ground green cardamom

- Vanilla extract

- Ground cinnamon

Instructions

1. Bring the butter to room temperature.

2. Roast the shredded coconut carefully until they turn a little brown.

3. Mix the butter, half of the coconut and spices.

4. Form into walnut-sized balls. Roll in the rest of the coconut.

5. Store in refrigerator or freezer.

Preparation Time: 5 minutes **Servings:** 1

Cooking Time: 10 minutes

Nutrition: Calories: 432 Protein: 23gFat: 3g Net Carbs: 5g

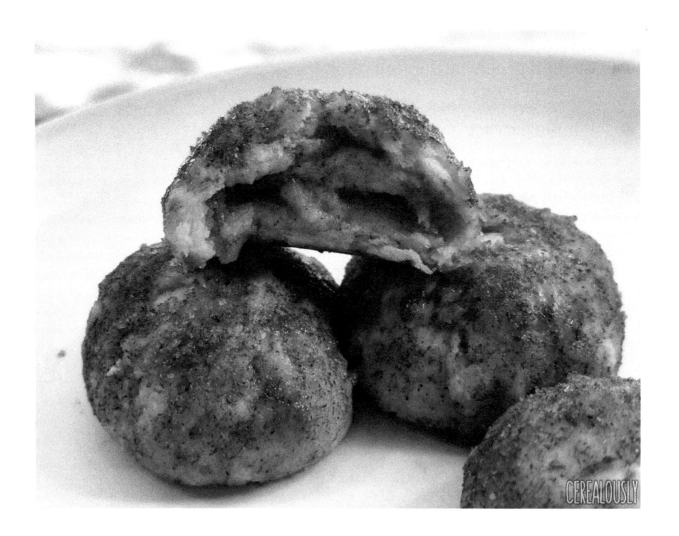

KETO CHEESECAKE AND BLUEBERRIES

Ingredients:

Crust:

- 1¼ cups almond flour

- 2 oz. butter

- 2 tbsp. erythritol

- ½ tsp vanilla extract

Filling:

- 20 oz. cream cheese

- ½ cup heavy whipping cream or crème fraiche

- 2 eggs

- 1 egg yolk

- 1 tsp lemon, zest

- ½ tsp vanilla extract

- 2 oz. fresh blueberries (optional)

Instructions

1. Preheat the oven to 350°F.

2. Butter a 9-inch springform and line the base of it with parchment paper.

3. Next, melt the butter for the crust and heat it until it lets off a nutty scent. This will give the crust an almost toffee-like flavor.

4. Remove it from the heat and add the almond flour, and vanilla. Combine these into firm dough and press the dough into the base of the pan. Bake for about 8 minutes, until the crust turns lightly golden. Set the crust aside and allow it to cool while you prepare the filling.

5. Combine together cream cheese, heavy cream, eggs, lemon zest, and the vanilla. Combine these ingredients well and make sure there are no lumps. Pour this cheese mixture over the crust.

6. Raise the heat of the oven to 400°F and bake for another 15 minutes.

7. Lower the heat to 230°F and bake for another 45-60 minutes.

8. Turn off the heat and let the dessert cool in the oven. Remove it when it has cooled completely and place it in the fridge to rest overnight. Serve it with fresh blueberries.

Preparation Time: 15 minutes **Servings:** 2

Cooking Time: 60 minutes

Nutrition: Calories: 158 Protein: 5g Fat: 8g Net Carbs: 21g

KETO GINGERBREAD CRÈME BRULE

Ingredients:

- 1¾ cups heavy whipping cream

- 2 tsp pumpkin pie spice

- 2 tbsp. erythritol (an all-natural sweetener)

- ¼ tsp vanilla extract

- 4 egg yolks

- ½ clementine (optional)

Instructions

1. Preheat the oven to 360°F.

2. Crack the eggs to separate them and place the egg whites and the egg yolks in two separate bowls. We will only use egg yolks in this recipe, so save the egg whites for a rainy day.

3. Add some cream to a saucepan and bring it to a boil along with the spices, vanilla extract, and sweetener mixed in.

4. Add the warm cream mixture into the egg yolks. Do this slowly, only adding a little bit at a time, while whisking.

5. Pour it into oven-proof ramekins or small Pyrex bowls that are firmly placed in a larger baking dish with large sides.

6. Add some water to the larger dish with the ramekins in it until it's about halfway up the ramekins. Make sure not to get water in the ramekins though. The water helps the cream cook gently and evenly for a creamy and smooth result.

7. Bake it in the oven for about 30 minutes. Take the ramekins out from the baking dish and let the dessert cool.

8. You can enjoy this dessert either warm or cold, you can also add a clementine segment on top of it.

Preparation Time: 15 minutes **Servings:** 6

Cooking Time: 30 minutes

Nutrition: Calories: 321 Protein: 14g Fat: 1g Net Carbs: 11 g

VEGETABLES

PORTOBELLO MUSHROOM PIZZA

Ingredients:

- 4 large Portobello mushrooms, stems removed

- ¼ cup olive oil

- 1 teaspoon minced garlic

- 1 medium tomato, cut into 4 slices

- 2 teaspoons chopped fresh basil

- 1 cup shredded mozzarella cheese

Instructions

- Preheat the oven to broil. Line a baking sheet with aluminum foil and set aside.

- In a small bowl, toss the mushroom caps with the olive oil until well coated. Use your fingertips to rub the oil in without breaking the mushrooms.

- Place the mushrooms on the baking sheet gill-side down and broil the mushrooms until they are tender on the tops, about 2 minute

- Flip the mushrooms over and broil 1 minute more

- Take the baking sheet out and spread the garlic over each mushroom, top each with a tomato slice, sprinkle with the basil, and top with the cheese

- Broil the mushrooms until the cheese is melted and bubbly, about 1 minute.

- Serve.

Preparation Time: 15 minutes **Servings:** 4

Cooking Time: 5 minutes

Nutrition: Calories: 251 Fat: 20g Protein: 14g Carbs: 7g Fiber: 3g Net Carbs: 4g Fat 71 Protein 19 Carbs 10

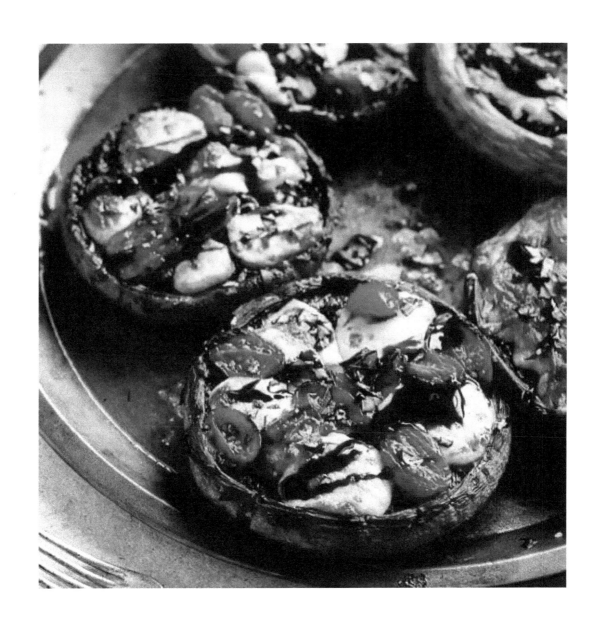

GARLICKY GREEN BEANS

Ingredients:

- 1 pound green beans, stemmed

- 2 tablespoons olive oil

- 1 teaspoon minced garlic

- Sea salt

- Freshly ground black pepper

- ¼ cup freshly grated Parmesan cheese

Instructions

1. Preheat the oven to 425°F. Line a baking sheet with aluminum foil and set aside.

2. In a large bowl, toss together the green beans, olive oil, and garlic until well mixed.

3. Season the beans lightly with salt and pepper

4. Spread the beans on the baking sheet and roast them until they are tender and lightly browned, stirring them once, about 10 minutes.

5. Serve topped with the Parmesan cheese.

Preparation Time: 10 minutes **Servings:** 4

Cooking Time: 10 minutes

Nutrition: Calories: 104 Fat: 9g Protein: 4g Carbs: 2g Fiber: 1g Net Carbs: 1g Fat 77 Protein 15 Carbs 8

SAUTÉED ASPARAGUS WITH WALNUTS

Ingredients:

- 1½ tablespoons olive oil

- ¾ pound asparagus, woody ends trimmed

- Sea salt

- Freshly ground pepper

- ¼ cup chopped walnuts

Directions:

1. Place a large skillet over medium-high heat and add the olive oil.

2. Sauté the asparagus until the spears are tender and lightly browned, about 5 minutes.

3. Season the asparagus with salt and pepper.

4. Remove the skillet from the heat and toss the asparagus with the walnuts.

5. Serve.

Preparation Time: 10 minutes **Servings:** 4

Cooking Time: 5 minutes

Nutrition: Calories: 124 Fat: 12g Protein: 3g Carbs: 4g Fiber: 2g Net Carbs: 2g Fat 81 Protein Carbs 10

BRUSSELS SPROUTS CASSEROLE

Ingredients:

- 8 bacon slices

- 1 pound Brussels sprouts, blanched for 10 minutes and cut into quarters

- 1 cup shredded Swiss cheese, divided

- ¾ cup heavy (whipping) cream

Instructions

1. Preheat the oven to 400°F.

2. Place a skillet over medium-high heat and cook the bacon until it is crispy, about 6 minutes.

3. Reserve 1 tablespoon of bacon fat to grease the casserole dish and roughly chop the cooked bacon.

4. Lightly oil a casserole dish with the reserved bacon fat and set aside.

5. In a medium bowl, toss the Brussels sprouts with the chopped bacon and ½ cup of cheese and transfer the mixture to the casserole dish.

6. Pour the heavy cream over the Brussels sprouts and top the casserole with the remaining ½ cup of cheese.

7. Bake until the cheese is melted and lightly browned and the vegetables are heated through, about 20 minutes.

8. Serve.

Preparation Time: 15 minutes **Servings:** 8

Cooking Time: 30 minutes

Nutrition: Calories: 299 Fat: 11g Protein: 12g Carbs: 7g Fiber: 3g Net Carbs: 4g Fat 77 Protein 15 Carbs 8

CREAMED SPINACH

Ingredients:

- 1 tablespoon butter

- ½ sweet onion, very thinly sliced

- 4 cups spinach, stemmed and thoroughly washed

- ¾ cup heavy (whipping) cream

- ¼ cup Herbed Chicken Stock

- Pinch sea salt

- Pinch freshly ground black pepper

- Pinch ground nutmeg

Instructions

1. In a large skillet over medium heat, add the butter.

2. Sauté the onion until it is lightly caramelized, about 5 minutes.

3. Stir in the spinach, heavy cream, chicken stock, salt, pepper, and nutmeg.

4. Sauté until the spinach is wilted, about 5 minutes.

5. Continue cooking the spinach until it is tender and the sauce is thickened, about 15 minutes.

6. Serve immediately.

Preparation Time: 10 minutes **Servings:** 4

Cooking Time: 30 minutes

Nutrition: Calories: 195 Fat: 20g Protein: 3g Carbs: 3g Fiber: 2g Net Carbs: 1g Fat 88 Protein 6 Carbs 6

CHEESY MASHED CAULIFLOWER

Ingredients:

- 1 head cauliflower, chopped roughly

- ½ cup shredded Cheddar cheese

- ¼ cup heavy (whipping) cream

- 2 tablespoons butter, at room temperature

- Sea salt

- Freshly ground black pepper

Instructions

1. Place a large saucepan filled three-quarters full with water over high heat and bring to a boil.

2. Blanch the cauliflower until tender, about 5 minutes, and drain.

3. Transfer the cauliflower to a food processor and add the cheese, heavy cream, and butter. Purée until very creamy and whipped.

4. Season with salt and pepper.

5. Serve.

Preparation Time: 15 minutes **Servings:** 4

Cooking Time: 5 minutes

Nutrition: Calories: 183 Fat: 15g Protein: 8g Carbs: 6g Fiber: 2g Net Carbs: 4g Fat 75 Protein 14 Carbs 11

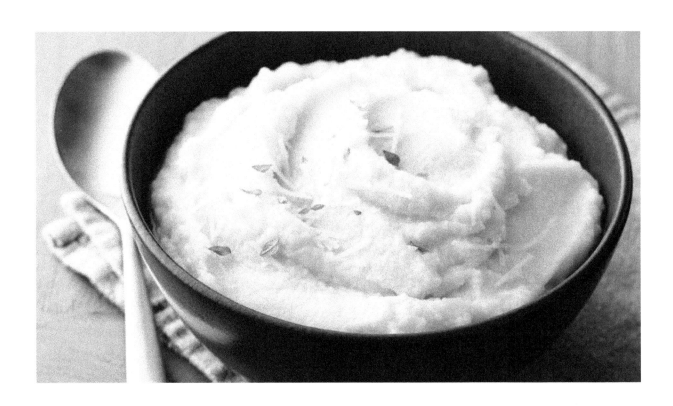

SAUTÉED CRISPY ZUCCHINI

Ingredients:

- 2 tablespoons butter

- 4 zucchini, cut into ¼-inch-thick rounds

- ½ cup freshly grated Parmesan cheese

- Freshly ground black pepper

Instructions

1. Place a large skillet over medium-high heat and melt the butter.

2. Add the zucchini and sauté until tender and lightly browned, about 5 minutes.

3. Spread the zucchini evenly in the skillet and sprinkle the Parmesan cheese over the vegetables.

4. Cook without stirring until the Parmesan cheese is melted and crispy where it touches the skillet, about 5 minutes.

5. Serve.

Preparation Time: 15 minutes **Servings:** 4

Cooking Time: 10 minutes

Nutrition: Calories: 94 Fat: 8g Protein: 4g Carbs: 1g Fiber: 0g Net Carbs: 1g Fat 76 Protein 20 Carbs 4

MUSHROOMS WITH CAMEMBERT

Ingredients:

- 2 tablespoons butter

- 2 teaspoons minced garlic

- 1 pound button mushrooms, halved

- 4 ounces Camembert cheese, diced

- Freshly ground black pepper

Instructions

1. Place a large skillet over medium-high heat and melt the butter.

2. Sauté the garlic until translucent, about 3 minutes.

3. Sauté the mushrooms until tender, about 10 minutes.

4. Stir in the cheese and sauté until melted, about 2 minutes.

5. Season with pepper and serve.

Preparation Time: 5 minutes **Servings:** 4

Cooking Time: 15 minutes

Nutrition: Calories: 161 Fat: 13g Protein: 9g Carbs: 4g Fiber: 1g Net Carbs: 3g Fat 70 Protein 21 Carbs 9

PESTO ZUCCHINI NOODLES

Ingredients:

- 4 small zucchini, ends trimmed

- ¾ cup Herb Kale Pesto ¼ cup grated or shredded

- Parmesan chees

Instructions

- Use a spiralizer or peeler to cut the zucchini into "noodles" and place them in a medium bowl.

- Add the pesto and the Parmesan cheese and toss to coat.

- Serve.

Preparation Time: 15 minutes **Servings:** 4

Cooking Time: 10 minutes

Nutrition: Calories: 93 Fat: 8g Protein: 4g Carbs: 2g Fiber: 0g Net Carbs: 2g Fat 70 Protein 15 Carbs 8

GOLDEN ROSTI

Ingredients:

- 8 bacon slices, chopped

- 1 cup shredded acorn squash

- 1 cup shredded raw celeriac

- 2 tablespoons grated or shredded Parmesan cheese

- 2 teaspoons minced garlic

- 1 teaspoon chopped fresh thyme

- Sea salt

- Freshly ground black pepper

- 2 tablespoons butter

Instructions

1. In a large skillet over medium-high heat, cook the bacon until crispy, about 5 minutes.

2. While the bacon is cooking, in a large bowl, mix together the squash, celeriac, Parmesan cheese, garlic, and thyme. Season the mixture generously with salt and pepper, and set aside.

3. Remove the cooked bacon with a slotted spoon to the rosti mixture and stir to incorporate.

4. Remove all but 2 tablespoons of bacon fat from the skillet and add the butter

5. Reduce the heat to medium-low and transfer the rosti mixture to the skillet and spread it out evenly to form a large round patty about 1 inch thick.

6. Cook until the bottom of the rosti is golden brown and crisp, about 5 minutes.

7. Flip the rosti over and cook until the other side is crispy and the middle is cooked through, about 5 minutes more.

8. Remove the skillet from the heat and cut the rosti into 8 pieces

9. Serve.

Preparation Time: 15 minutes **Servings:** 8

Cooking Time: 15 minutes

Nutrition: Calories: 171 Fat: 15g Protein: 5g Carbs: 3g Fiber: 0g Net Carbs: 3g Fat 81 Protein 12 Carbs 7

ARTICHOKE AND AVOCADO PASTA SALAD

Ingredients:

- Two cups of spiral pasta (uncooked)

- A quarter cup of Romano cheese (grated)

- One can (fourteen oz.) of artichoke hearts (coarsely chopped and drained well)

- One avocado (medium-sized, ripe, cubed)

- Two plum tomatoes (chopped coarsely)

For the dressing:

- One tbsp. of fresh cilantro (chopped)

- Two tbsps. of lime juice

- A quarter cup of canola oil

- One and a half tsps. of lime zest (grated)

- Half a tsp. each of

- Pepper (freshly ground)

- Kosher salt

Instructions

1. Follow the directions mentioned on the package for cooking the pasta. Drain them well and rinse using cold water.

2. Then, take a large-sized bowl and in it, add the pasta along with the tomatoes, artichoke hearts, cheese, and avocado. Combine them well. Then, take another bowl and add all the ingredients of the dressing in it. Whisk them together and, once combined, add the dressing over the pasta.

3. Gently toss the mixture to coat everything evenly in the dressing and then refrigerate.

Preparation Time: 15 minutes **Servings:** 10 servings

Cooking Time: 30 minutes

Nutrition: Calories: 188 Protein: 6g Fat: 10g Carbs: 21g Fiber: 2g

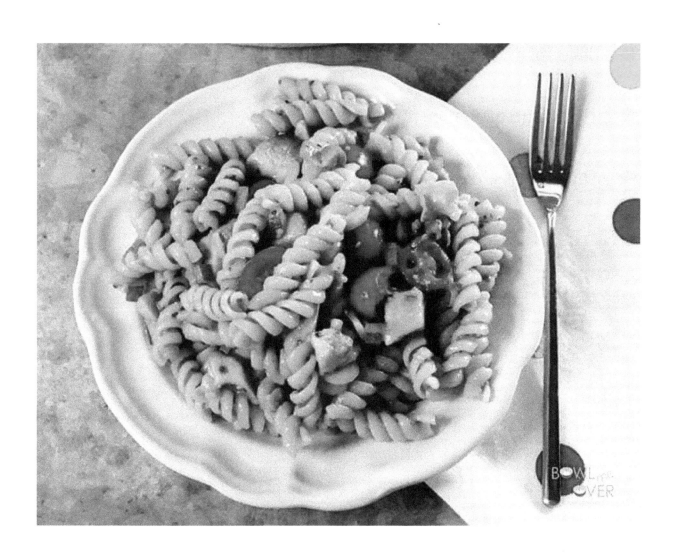

109

APPLE ARUGULA AND TURKEY SALAD IN A JAR

Ingredients:

- Three tbsps. of red wine vinegar

- Two tbsps. of chives (freshly minced)

- Half a cup of orange juice

- One to three tbsps. of sesame oil

- A quarter tsp. each of

- Pepper (coarsely ground)

- Salt

For the salad:

- Four tsps. of curry powder

- Four cups each of

- Turkey (cubed, cooked)

- Baby spinach or fresh arugula

- A quarter tsp. of salt

- Half a tsp. of pepper (coarsely ground)

- One cup of halved green grapes

- One apple (large-sized, chopped)

- Eleven oz. of mandarin oranges (properly drained)

- One tbsp. of lemon juice

- Half a cup each of

- Walnuts (chopped)

- Dried cranberries or pomegranate seeds

Instructions

- Take a small-sized bowl and, in it, add the first 6 ingredients from the list into it. Whisk them. Then take a large bowl and in it, add the turkey and then add the seasonings on top of it. Toss the turkey cubes to coat them with the seasoning. Take another bowl and in it, add the lemon juice and toss the apple chunks in the juice.

- Take four jars and divide the layers in the order I mention here - first goes the orange juice mixture, the second layer is that of the turkey, then apple, oranges, grapes, cranberries or pomegranate seeds, walnuts, and spinach or arugula. Cover the jars and then refrigerate them.

Preparation Time: 10 minutes **Servings:** 4 servings

Cooking Time: 10 minutes

Nutrition: Calories: 471 Protein: 45g Fat: 19g Carbs: 33g Fiber: 5g

SUMMERTIME SLAW

Ingredients:

- One-third cup of canola oil

- Three-quarter cups each of

- White vinegar

- Sugar

- One tsp. each of

- Pepper

- Salt

- One tbsp. of water

- Half a tsp. of red pepper flakes (crushed and optional)

- Two tomatoes (medium-sized, seeded, peeled, and chopped)

- One pack of coleslaw mix (fourteen oz.)

- One sweet red pepper (small-sized, chopped)

- One green pepper (small-sized, chopped)

- One onion (large-sized, chopped)

- Half a cup of sweet pickle relish

Instructions

1. Take a saucepan of large size and in it, combine water, sugar, oil, vinegar, pepper, salt, and if you want, then red pepper flakes too. Cook them over medium heat by continuously stirring the mixture. Keep stirring until it comes to a boil. Cook for another two minutes or so and make sure that all the sugar has dissolved. Once done, cool the mixture to room temperature by stirring it.

2. Take a salad bowl of large size and in it, combine the pickle relish, coleslaw mix, peppers, onion, and tomatoes. On top of the mixture, add the dressing and toss the mixture to coat it properly. Cover the mixture and put it in the refrigerator for a night.

Preparation Time: 20 minutes **Servings:** 10-12

Cooking Time: 30 minutes

Nutrition: Calories: 138 Protein: 1g Fat: 6g Carbs: 21g Fiber: 2g

ZUCCHINI AND TOMATO SPAGHETTI

Ingredients:

- Two large-sized zucchini nicely spiralizer

- Three cups of red and yellow cherry tomatoes

- Four oz. of spaghetti (whole wheat – optional)

- Toppings – grated parmesan

For the avocado sauce:

- A quarter cup of olive oil

- One avocado

- Half a cup of parsley (fresh)

- Half a tsp. of salt

- Three-four green onions (only the green parts)

- One lemon (juiced)

- One clove of garlic

- A pinch of pepper (freshly ground)

Instructions

1. Firstly, take all the ingredients of the sauce and pulse them so that they are combined well and form a smooth mixture. Set it aside.

2. Then, follow the directions mentioned in the package for cooking the spaghetti. Drain the cooked spaghetti and keep it aside too.

3. Take a large-sized skillet and heat the cherry tomatoes in it. Use a bit of olive oil. Keep cooking the tomatoes until they seem well-roasted, and they will also seem loosened with their skins split. Once done, remove the tomatoes from the flame and set it aside.

4. Then, add the zucchini to the same skillet. Stir and toss them for about two minutes until they look crisp. Then, add the avocado sauce and the spaghetti. Keep tossing until everything has properly combined. Season with pepper and salt as per taste. Top with parmesan and the tomatoes that you had reserved earlier.

Preparation Time: 10 minutes **Servings:** 4 servings

Cooking Time: 20 minutes

Nutrition: Calories: 330 Protein: 7.1g Fat: 20g Carbs: 35.3g Fiber: 8g

WHITE BEAN SALAD

Ingredients:

For the salad:

- Two green peppers coarsely chopped

- Half a cup each of

- Chopped cucumber

- Chopped tomatoes

- One and a half cups of white beans (boiled)

- A quarter cup each of

- Green onions (chopped)

- Fresh dill (chopped)

- Parsley (chopped)

- Four eggs (hard-boiled)

For the dressing:

- One tbsp. of lemon juice

- One tsp. of vinegar

- Two tbsps. of olive oil

- One tsp. of sumac

- Half a tsp. of salt

- For quick onion pickle,

- One tsp. each of

- Sumac

- Salt

- Vinegar

- One tbsp. of lemon juice

- Two thinly sliced red onions (medium-sized)

- Two cups of water (hot)

Instructions

1. Take a large-sized bowl and add all the salad ingredients in it, but keep the eggs aside.

2. In case you do not want to pickle the onions, you can simply make thin slices and then mix them with the other ingredients. But, if you do want to pickle the onions, then continue with it before you move on to the dressing. The recipe for the onions is mentioned later.

3. Take all the ingredients of the dressing together in one bowl and whisk them together. Then, drizzle the dressing over the salad. Toss well, and on the top, place halved eggs.

For the pickled onions:

- First, take very hot water and place the sliced onions in it. Blanch the onions for one minute and then immediately transfer them into a pot of very cold water so that the cooking stops. Let them stay in that pot of cold water for a few minutes. Once done, drain them well.

- Mix sumac, lemon juice, salt, and vinegar together and then pour the mixture over the onion that you just drained. Keep it for five to ten minutes.

- Then, add the onions into the mixture of salad and stir well. Keep some onions aside so that you can use them as a topping.

Preparation Time: 5 minutes **Servings:** 4 servings

Cooking Time: 10 minutes

Nutrition: Calories: 449 Protein: 23.6g Fat: 23.3g Carbs: 39.7g

LENTIL BOLOGNESE

Ingredients:

- Two boxes of penne pasta

- One onion (medium-sized, finely chopped)

- One red bell pepper (finely chopped)

- Two tbsps. of olive oil

- Two carrots (large-sized, sliced)

- Four cloves of garlic (large ones, minced)

- One tbsp. of miso

- One tsp. each of

- Pepper

- Salt

- Four cups of water

- One can of tomato paste (measuring five and a half ounces)

- One cup each of

- Brown lentils (dried)

- Cherry tomatoes (halved)

- Toppings (optional) – black pepper, sage leaves, parmesan (grated)

Instructions

1. Take a large-sized skillet and start by heating the oil in it on medium flame. Then, add the chopped onions. In about five minutes, they will soften and appear to be translucent. Then, add the red pepper, carrots, sugar, and sea salt to the skillet and keep cooking. Stir the mixture from time to time. In fifteen minutes, everything will be well caramelized. Then, add the tomato paste and the garlic and let the mixture cook for three minutes or until you get a caramelized fragrance from the paste.

2. Then, add the lentils, miso, and water to the skillet and bring the mixture to a boil. Once the mixture is boiling, reduce the

flame and keep the skillet uncovered while the lentils are cooking. This will take about twenty-five to thirty minutes. Keep stirring the lentils from time to time, and in case they look dry, add some water. After that, add the cherry tomatoes and keep stirring.

3. While you are cooking the lentils, take a large pot and fill it with water. Add generous amounts of salt and bring the water to a boil. Then, add the chickpea pasta into the water and cook it for about five to six minutes or until al dente. Don't overcook it. Once done, drain the water and set them aside to cool.

4. Divide the penne into four to six meal prep containers and top with Bolognese. Sprinkle a few sage leaves or a bit of parmesan if you want.

Preparation Time: 20 minutes **Servings:** 4-6 servings

Cooking Time: 40 minutes

Nutrition: Calories: 486 Protein: 29.3g Fat: 9g Carbs: 78.2g Fiber: 15g

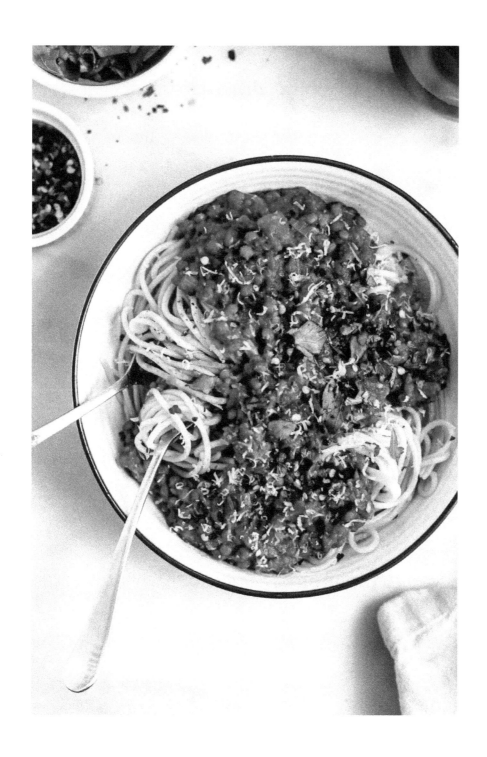

KALE, LEMON, AND WHITE BEAN SOUP

Ingredients:

- One hundred fifty grams of dried cannellini beans

- Two cups of vegetable stock

- Five cups of water

- One white onion (large-sized, diced)

- Two tbsps. of olive oil

- Eight cloves of garlic

- Kombu (one-inch strip)

- One tsp. of dried thyme

- Two potatoes (small ones, cubed after peeling)

- Two bay leaves

- One cup of kale

- One lemon (juiced and zest)

Instructions

- Take an ample amount of water to soak the dried beans and keep them soaked for about twelve hours. Drain the beans properly and they should become double their size. Rinse them and they are ready to be cooked.

- Take a large-sized pot, and in it, add one tbsp. of oil and heat it. Then, add the diced onion in the pot and cook the onions until they become golden and soft.

- Then, add the stock and water along with garlic, dried beans, kombu, thyme, and bay leaves. Keep the pot covered and then bring it to a boil. Once it starts boiling, reduce the flame to a simmer and wait for about forty minutes.

- While it is cooking, start with the kale. Wash it thoroughly. All the inner stalks that are tough should be removed. Then, start slicing them into ribbons of one-inch each. It looks good when you have delicate small pieces, so you should take your time with this.

- After about half an hour, add the potatoes to the pot and then let the preparation simmer for ten more minutes. After this, both the potatoes and the beans should be soft. Take out the kombu and bay leaves. Take a potato masher and use it carefully to mash at least half of the beans and potatoes.

- Add the kale. Cook the mixture for ten more minutes. The water content needs to be checked now and see whether it is right or whether it needs to be topped up a bit. If the water is too much, then cook uncovered for a few minutes so that it dries up.

- Once you notice the kale softening, take a tbsp. of olive oil and add it to the pot. Stir in the zest and lemon juice as well, and your dish is ready.

Preparation Time: 20 minutes **Servings:** 2 servings

Cooking Time: 1 hour 10 minutes

Nutrition: Calories: 574 Protein: 22g Fat: 16g Carbs: 106g Fiber: 23g

ALOO GOBI

Ingredients:

- 1 large cauliflower, cut into 1-inch pieces

- 1 large russet potato, peeled and diced

- 1 medium yellow onion, peeled and diced

- 1 cup canned diced tomatoes, with juice

- 1 cup frozen peas

- ¼ cup water

- 1 (2-inch) piece fresh ginger, peeled and finely chopped

- 1½ teaspoons minced garlic (3 cloves)

- 1 jalapeño pepper, stemmed and sliced

- 1 tablespoon cumin seeds

- 1 tablespoon garam masala

- 1 teaspoon ground turmeric

- 1 heaping tablespoon fresh cilantro

- Cooked rice, for serving (optional)

Instructions

1. Combine the cauliflower, potato, onion, diced tomatoes, peas, water, ginger, garlic, jalapeño, cumin seeds, garam masala, and turmeric in a slow cooker; mix until well combined.

2. Cover and cook on low for 4 to 5 hours.

3. Garnish with the cilantro, and serve over cooked rice (if using).

Preparation Time: 15 Minutes **Servings:** 4

Cooking Time: 4 To 5 Hours

Nutrition: Calories: 115 Total fat: 1g Protein: 6g Sodium: 62mg Fiber: 6g

JACKFRUIT CARNITAS

Ingredients:

- 2 (20-ounce) cans jackfruit, drained, hard pieces discarded

- ¾ cup Very Easy Vegetable Broth or store bought

- 1 tablespoon ground cumin

- 1 tablespoon dried oregano

- 1½ teaspoons ground coriander

- 1 teaspoon minced garlic (2 cloves)

- ½ teaspoon ground cinnamon

- 2 bay leaves

- Tortillas, for serving

- Optional toppings: diced onions, sliced radishes, fresh cilantro, lime wedges, Nacho Cheese

Instructions

- Combine the jackfruit, vegetable broth, cumin, oregano, coriander, garlic, cinnamon, and bay leaves in a slow cooker. Stir to combine.

- Cover and cook on low for 8 hours or on high for 4 hours.

- Use two forks to pull the jackfruit apart into shreds.

- Remove the bay leaves. Serve in warmed tortillas with your favorite taco fixings.

Preparation Time: 15 Minutes **Servings:** 4

Cooking Time: 8 Hours

Nutrition: Calories: 286 Total fat: 2g Protein: 6g Sodium: 155mg Fiber: 5g

BAKED BEANS

Ingredients:

- 2 (15-ounce) cans white beans, drained and rinsed

- 1 (15-ounce) can tomato sauce

- 1 medium yellow onion, finely diced

- 1½ teaspoons minced garlic (3 cloves)

- 3 tablespoons brown sugar

- 2 tablespoons molasses

- 1 tablespoon prepared yellow mustard

- 1 tablespoon chili powder

- 1 teaspoon soy sauce

- Pinch salt

- Freshly ground black pepper

Instructions

1. Place the beans, tomato sauce, onion, garlic, brown sugar, molasses, mustard, chili powder, and soy sauce into a slow cooker; mix well.

2. Cover and cook on low for 6 hours. Season with salt and pepper before serving.

Preparation Time: 15 Minutes **Servings:** 4

Cooking Time: 6 Hours

Nutrition: Calories: 468 Total fat: 2g Protein: 28g Sodium: 714mg Fiber: 20g

BRUSSELS SPROUTS CURRY

Ingredients:

- ¾ pound Brussels sprouts, bottoms cut off and sliced in half

- 1 can full-fat coconut milk

- 1 cup Very Easy Vegetable Broth or store bought

- 1 medium onion, diced

- 1 medium carrot, thinly sliced

- 1 medium red or Yukon potato, diced

- 1½ teaspoons minced garlic (3 cloves)

- 1 (1-inch) piece fresh ginger, peeled and minced

- 1 small serrano chili, seeded and finely chopped

- 2 tablespoons peanut butter

- 1 tablespoon rice vinegar or other vinegar

- 1 tablespoon cane sugar or agave nectar

- 1 tablespoon soy sauce

- 1 teaspoon curry powder

- 1 teaspoon ground turmeric

- Pinch salt

- Freshly ground black pepper

- Cooked rice, for serving (optional)

Instructions

1. Place the Brussels sprouts, coconut milk, vegetable broth, onion, carrot, potato, garlic, ginger, serrano chili, peanut butter, vinegar, cane sugar, soy sauce, curry powder, and turmeric in a slow cooker. Mix well.

2. Cover and cook on low for 7 to 8 hours or on high for 4 to 5 hours.

3. Season with salt and pepper. Serve over rice (if using).

Preparation Time: 15 Minutes **Servings:** 4

Cooking Time: 7 To 8 Hours

Nutrition: Calories: 404 Total fat: 29g Protein: 10g

Sodium: 544mg Fiber: 8g

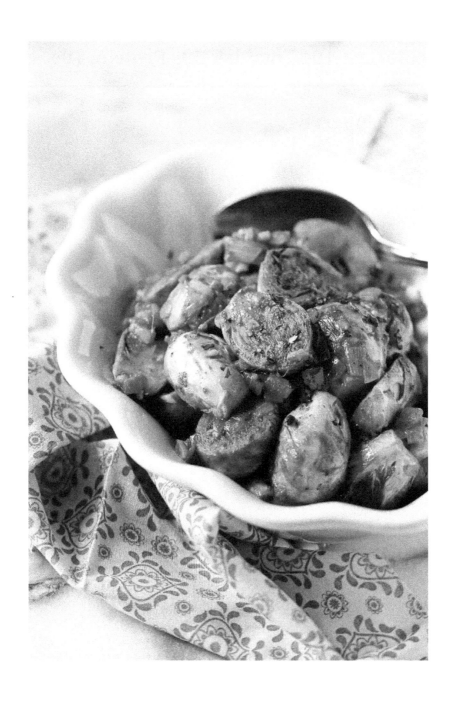

JAMBALAYA

Ingredients:

- 2 cups Very Easy Vegetable Broth or store bought

- 1 large yellow onion, diced

- 1 green bell pepper, seeded and chopped

- 2 celery stalks, chopped

- 1½ teaspoons minced garlic (3 cloves)

- 1 (15-ounce) can dark red kidney beans, drained and rinsed

- 1 (15-ounce) can black-eyed peas, drained and rinsed

- 1 (15-ounce) can diced tomatoes, drained

- 2 tablespoons Cajun seasoning

- 2 teaspoons dried oregano

- 2 teaspoons dried parsley

- 1 teaspoon cayenne pepper

- 1 teaspoon smoked paprika

- ½ teaspoon dried thyme

- Cooked rice, for serving (optional)

Instructions

1. Combine the vegetable broth, onion, bell pepper, celery, garlic, kidney beans, black-eyed peas, diced tomatoes, Cajun seasoning, oregano, parsley, cayenne pepper, smoked paprika, and dried thyme in a slow cooker; mix well.

2. Cover and cook on low for 6 to 8 hours.

3. Serve over rice (if using).

Preparation Time: 15 Minutes **Servings:** 4

Cooking Time: 6 To 8 Hours

Nutrition: Calories: 428 Total fat: 2g Protein: 28g Sodium: 484mg Fiber: 19g

MUSHROOM-KALE STROGANOFF

Ingredients:

- 1 pound mushrooms, sliced

- 1½ cups Very Easy Vegetable Broth or store bought

- 1 cup stemmed and chopped kale

- 1 small yellow onion, diced

- 2 garlic cloves, minced

- 2 tablespoons all-purpose flour

- 2 tablespoons ketchup or tomato paste

- 2 teaspoons paprika

- ½ cup vegan sour cream

- ¼ cup chopped fresh parsley

- Cooked rice, pasta, or quinoa, for serving

Instructions

- Combine the mushrooms, vegetable broth, kale, onion, garlic, flour, ketchup or tomato paste, and paprika in a slow cooker. Mix thoroughly.

- Cover and cook on low for 6 to 8 hours.

- Stir in the sour cream and parsley just before serving.

- Serve over rice, pasta, or quinoa.

Preparation Time: 15 Minutes **Servings:** 4

Cooking Time: 6 To 8 Hours

Nutrition: Calories: 146 Total fat: 7g Protein: 8g Sodium: 417mg Fiber: 3g

SLOPPY JOE FILLING

Ingredients:

- 3 cups textured vegetable protein

- 3 cups water

- 2 (6-ounce) cans tomato paste, or 1 cup ketchup

- 1 medium yellow onion, diced

- ½ medium green bell pepper, finely diced

- 2 teaspoons minced garlic (4 cloves)

- 4 tablespoons vegan Worcestershire sauce

- 3 tablespoons brown sugar

- 3 tablespoons apple cider vinegar

- 3 tablespoons prepared yellow mustard

- 2 tablespoons hot sauce (optional)

- 1 tablespoon salt

- 1 teaspoon chili powder

- Sliced, toasted buns or cooked rice, for serving

Instructions

- Combine the textured vegetable protein, water, tomato paste, onion, bell pepper, garlic, Worcestershire sauce, brown sugar, vinegar, mustard, hot sauce (if using), salt, and chili powder in a slow cooker. Mix well.

- Cover and cook on low for 6 to 8 hours or on high for 4 to 5 hours.

- Serve on sliced, toasted buns or over rice.

Preparation Time: 15 Minutes **Servings:** 4

Cooking Time: 6 To 8 Hours

Nutrition: Calories: 452 Total fat: 4g Protein: 75g Sodium: 2,242mg Fiber: 11g

HOPPIN' JOHN

Ingredients:

- 3 (15-ounce) cans black-eyed peas, drained and rinsed

- 1 (14.5-ounce) can Cajun-style stewed tomatoes, with juice

- 2 cups hot water

- 1 cup stemmed and chopped kale

- ¾ cup finely diced red bell pepper

- ½ cup sliced scallions

- 1 medium jalapeño pepper, seeded and minced

- 1 teaspoon minced garlic (2 cloves)

- 1½ teaspoons hot sauce

- 1 vegetable bouillon cube

- Cooked rice, for serving

Instructions

1. Combine the black-eyed peas, tomatoes, hot water, kale, bell pepper, scallions, jalapeño, garlic, hot sauce, and bouillon cube in a slow cooker. Stir to combine.

2. Cover and cook on low for 4 to 6 hours.

3. Serve over cooked rice.

Preparation Time: 15 Minutes **Servings:** 4

Cooking Time: 4 To 6 Hours

Nutrition: Calories: 164 Total fat: 2g Protein: 10g Sodium: 250mg Fiber: 8g

AFRICAN SWEET POTATO STEW

Ingredients:

- 4 cups peeled diced sweet potatoes

- 1 (15-ounce) can red kidney beans, drained and rinsed

- 1 (14.5-ounce) can diced tomatoes, drained

- 1 cup diced red bell pepper

- 2 cups Very Easy Vegetable Broth or store bought

- 1 medium yellow onion, chopped

- 1 (4.5-ounce) can chopped green chilies, drained

- 1 teaspoon minced garlic (2 cloves)

- 1½ teaspoons ground ginger

- 1 teaspoon ground cumin

- 4 tablespoons creamy peanut butter

- Pinch salt

- Freshly ground black pepper

Instructions

1. Combine the sweet potatoes, kidney beans, diced tomatoes, bell pepper, vegetable broth, onion, green chilies, garlic, ginger, and cumin in a slow cooker. Mix well

2. Cover and cook on low for 7 to 8 hours.

3. Ladle a little of the soup into a small bowl and mix in the peanut butter, then pour the mixture back into the stew

4. Season with salt and pepper. Mix well and serve.

Preparation Time: 15 Minutes **Servings:** 4

Cooking Time: 7 To 8 Hours

Nutrition: Calories: 514 Total fat: 10g Protein: 22g Sodium: 649mg Fiber: 17g

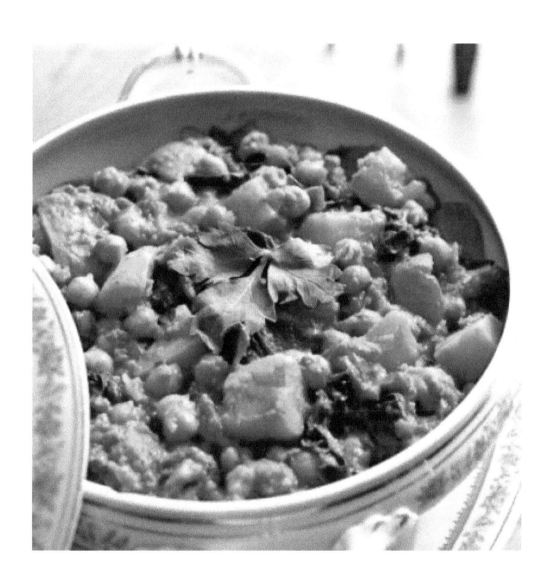

149

SWEET-AND-SOUR TEMPEH

Ingredients:

For The Sauce:

- ¾ cup fresh or canned pineapple chunks

- ½ cup crushed tomatoes

- ½ cup water

- ¼ cup chopped onion

- ¼ cup soy sauce

- 2 tablespoons rice vinegar

- ¼ teaspoon red pepper flakes

- 1 (½-inch) piece fresh ginger, peeled

For The Tempeh:

- 2 (8-ounce) packages tempeh, cut into cubes

- 2 cups diced bell pepper

- 1½ cups diced pineapple

- ½ cup diced onion

- Cooked rice, for serving

Instructions

1. Put the pineapple chunks, crushed tomatoes, water, onion, soy sauce, rice vinegar, red pepper flakes, and ginger in a blender; blend until smooth.

2. Combine the sauce, tempeh, bell pepper, diced pineapple, and onion in a slow cooker; stir well.

3. Cover and cook on low for 7 to 8 hours.

4. Serve over cooked rice.

Preparation Time: 15 Minutes **Servings:** 4

Cooking Time: 7 To 8 Hours

Nutrition: Calories: 324 Total fat: 13g Protein: 24g Sodium: 974mg Fiber: 4g

JACKFRUIT COCHINITA PIBIL

Ingredients:

- 2 (20-ounce) cans jackfruit, drained, hard pieces discarded

- 2/3 cup freshly squeezed lemon juice

- 1/3 cup orange juice

- 2 habanero peppers, seeded and chopped

- 2 tablespoons achiote paste

- 2 teaspoons ground cumin

- 2 teaspoons smoked paprika

- 2 teaspoons chili powder

- 2 teaspoons ground coriander

- Pinch salt

- Freshly ground black pepper

- Warmed corn tortillas, for serving

Instructions

- Combine the jackfruit, lemon juice, orange juice, habanero peppers, achiote paste, cumin, smoked paprika, chili powder, and coriander in a slow cooker; mix well.

- Cover and cook on low for 8 hours or on high for 4 hours.

- Use two forks to pull the jackfruit apart into shreds. Season with salt and pepper.

- Heat tortillas directly over a gas fire, or in a skillet over medium heat for about 1 minute per side. Spoon the jackfruit into the tortillas and serve.

Preparation Time: 15 Minutes **Servings:** 4

Cooking Time: 8 Hours

Nutrition: Calories: 297 Total fat: 2g Protein: 5g Sodium: 71mg Fiber: 6g

DELIGHTFUL DAL

Ingredients:

- 3 cups red lentils, rinsed

- 6 cups water

- 1 (28-ounce) can diced tomatoes, with juice

- 1 small yellow onion, diced

- 2½ teaspoons minced garlic (5 cloves)

- 1 (1-inch) piece fresh ginger, peeled and minced

- 1 tablespoon ground turmeric

- 2 teaspoons ground cumin

- 1½ teaspoons ground cardamom

- 1½ teaspoons whole mustard seeds

- 1 teaspoon fennel seeds

- 1 bay leaf

- 1 teaspoon salt

- ¼ teaspoon freshly ground black pepper

Instructions

1. Combine the lentils, water, diced tomatoes, onion, garlic, ginger, turmeric, cumin, cardamom, mustard seeds, fennel seeds, bay leaf, salt, and pepper in a slow cooker; mix well.

2. Cover and cook on low for 7 to 9 hours or on high for 4 to 6 hours.

3. Remove the bay leaf, and serve.

Preparation Time: 15 Minutes **Servings:** 4

Cooking Time: 7 To 9 Hours

Nutrition: Calories: 585 Total fat: 4g Protein: 40g Sodium: 616mg Fiber: 48g

MOROCCAN CHICKPEA STEW

Ingredients:

- 1 small butternut squash, peeled and chopped into bite-size pieces

- 3 cups Very Easy Vegetable Broth or store bought

- 1 medium yellow onion, diced

- 1 bell pepper, diced

- 1 (15-ounce) can chickpeas, drained and rinsed

- 1 (14.5-ounce) can tomato sauce

- ¾ cup brown lentils, rinsed

- 1½ teaspoons minced garlic (3 cloves)

- 1½ teaspoons ground ginger

- 1½ teaspoons ground turmeric

- 1½ teaspoons ground cumin

- 1 teaspoon ground cinnamon

- ¾ teaspoon smoked paprika

- ½ teaspoon salt

- 1 (8-ounce) package fresh udon noodles

- Freshly ground black pepper

Instructions

1. Combine the butternut squash, vegetable broth, onion, bell pepper, chickpeas, tomato sauce, brown lentils, garlic, ginger, turmeric, cumin, cinnamon, smoked paprika, and salt in a slow cooker. Mix well.

2. Cover and cook 6 to 8 hours on low or 3 to 4 hours on high. In the last 10 minutes of cooking, add the noodles.

3. Season with pepper, and serve.

Preparation Time: 15 Minutes **Servings:** 4

Cooking Time: 6 To 8 Hours

Nutrition: Calories: 427 Total fat: 4g Protein: 26g Sodium: 1,423mg Fiber: 24g

BROCCOLI QUINOA CASSEROLE

Ingredients:

- Four and a half cups of vegetable stock

- Two and a half cups of quinoa (uncooked)

- Half a tsp. of salt

- Two tablespoons of pesto sauce

- Two teaspoons of cornstarch

- Twelve ounces of mozzarella cheese (skimmed)

- Two cups of spinach (fresh and organic)

- One-third cup of parmesan cheese

- Three medium-sized green onions (chopped)

- Twelve ounces of broccoli florets (fresh)

Instructions

1. Set the temperature of the oven to 400 degrees Fahrenheit and preheat. Take a rectangular baking dish and add the quinoa to it along with the green onions. In the meantime, take a large-sized bowl and add the broccoli florets to it. Microwave the florets at high for about five minutes. Once done, set them aside.

2. Take a large-sized mixing bowl and in it, add the pesto, vegetable sauce, cornstarch, and salt. Use a wire whisk to mix all of them properly. Now, heat this mixture until it starts to boil. You can either do this in the microwave, or you can use your stovetop as well.

3. Now, take the vegetable stock and the spinach and add them to the quinoa. Add the three-quarter of the mozzarella cheese and the parmesan as well. Bake the mixture for thirty to thirty-five minutes. Once done, take the casserole of quinoa out and then mix the broccoli into it. Take the rest of the cheese and sprinkle on top. Place the preparation back in the oven for another five minutes. By this time, all the cheese will melt.

Preparation Time: 15 minutes **Servings:** 5

Cooking Time: 30 minutes

Nutrition: Calories: 49 Protein: 27.6g Fat: 16g Carbs: 61.3g Fiber: 9g

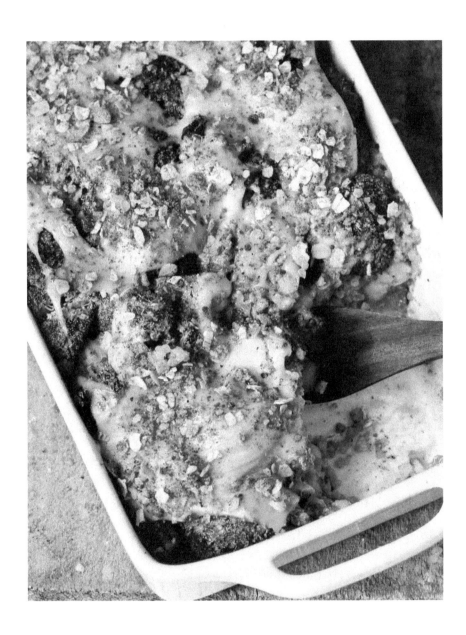

RATATOUILLE

Ingredients:

- 3 cups peeled diced eggplant

- 1 medium yellow onion, thinly sliced

- 1 green bell pepper, cut into strips

- 1 red bell pepper, cut into strips

- 3 medium zucchini, sliced

- 2 teaspoons minced garlic (4 cloves)

- 1½ (28-ounce) cans plum tomatoes, drained

- 3 tablespoons tomato paste

- 2½ tablespoons olive oil

- Pinch salt, plus more for salting eggplant

- Freshly ground black pepper

- ½ cup chopped fresh basil, for garnish

Instructions

1. Put the diced eggplant in a colander over the sink, sprinkle with salt, and set aside.

2. Put the onion, bell peppers, zucchini, and garlic in a slow cooker. Pat the eggplant dry and stir it into the slow cooker.

3. Add the tomatoes, tomato paste, and olive oil to the slow cooker and mix thoroughly.

4. Cover and cook on low for 6 hours.

5. Season with salt and pepper. Garnish with the basil and serve.

Preparation Time: 15 Minutes **Servings:** 4

Cooking Time: 6 Hours

Nutrition: Calories: 226 Total fat: 10g Protein: 7g Sodium: 85mg Fiber: 7g

CAULIFLOWER BOLOGNESE

Ingredients:

- ½ head cauliflower, cut into florets

- 1 (8- to 10-ounce) container button mushrooms

- 1 small yellow onion, quartered

- 2 medium carrots, scrubbed and cut into chunks

- 2 cups eggplant chunks

- 2½ teaspoons minced garlic (5 cloves)

- 2 (28-ounce) cans crushed tomatoes

- 2 tablespoons tomato paste

- 2 tablespoons cane sugar or agave nectar

- 2 tablespoons balsamic vinegar

- 2 tablespoons nutritional yeast

- 1½ tablespoons dried oregano

- 1½ tablespoons dried basil

- 1½ teaspoons chopped fresh rosemary leaves

- Pinch salt

- Freshly ground black pepper

Instructions

1. In a food processor, pulse the cauliflower, mushrooms, onion, carrots, eggplant, and garlic, until all the vegetables are finely chopped. Transfer to a slow cooker.

2. Add the crushed tomatoes, tomato paste, cane sugar, balsamic vinegar, nutritional yeast, oregano, basil, and rosemary to the slow cooker; mix well.

3. Cover and cook on low for 8 to 9 hours or on high for 4 to 5 hours.

4. Season with salt and pepper, and serve.

Preparation Time: 15 Minutes **Servings:** 4

Cooking Time: 8 To 9 Hours

Nutrition: Calories: 281 Total fat: 10g Protein: 17g Sodium: 855mg Fiber: 20g

CONCLUSION

We have reached the end of this wonderful journey, I hope you found it easy to prepare these recipes, you will see that with time, they will become very easy, you just need to train and you will become a star chef.

I would like to remind you that every time you start a diet or change your nutritional plan, it is always better to consult a nutritionist who can accompany you on your journey.

Thank you and I embrace you.

Lightning Source UK Ltd.
Milton Keynes UK
UKHW050913260421
382633UK00002B/58